DEDICATION

This book is dedicated to all those with challenges of mental disorders to the strengths and unique perspectives of neurodivergent individuals. There is new hope my friend.

Contents

Promoting mental well-being among colleagues and employees 1

DEDICATION 3

INTRODUCTION 5

CHAPTER ONE 6

CHAPTER TWO 10

CHAPTER THREE 13

CHAPTER FOUR 17

    The Intersection of Outcome Regret and Mental Health. 17

CHAPTER FIVE 23

    Fundraising Strategies for Mental Health Care. 23

CHAPTER SIX 29

    General well-being first. 29

CHAPTER SEVEN 34

    The link between emotional well-being and mental disorders. .. 34

CHAPTER EIGHT 38

    How Mental Health Startups Are Changing Lives: Overcoming Challenges: Regulation and Ethics in Mental Health Startups. 38

CHAPTER NINE 43

    Sharing personal experiences on a mental health blog. 43

CHAPTER TEN 46

Mental Health and Wellbeing at workplace

Promoting mental well-being among colleagues and employees

Dr. Martin Dosh

Copyright © 2022 CP Print all rights reserved

The characters and events portrayed in this book are fictitious. Any similarity to real persons, living or dead is coincidental and not intended by the author.

No part of this book may be reproduced, or stored in a retrieval system, or transmitted in any form or by any means, electronic, mechanical, photocopying, recording, or otherwise, without express written permission of the publisher.

ISBN: 9798325355899
Imprint: Independently published

Cover design by: Art Painter Librar Congress Control Number: 2018675309

Printed in the United States of America

Addressing mental health in residential care. 46

CHAPTER ELEVEN 52

CHAPTER TWELVE 57

Creating Authentic and Compassionate Messages 57

CHAPTER THIRETEEN 61

CHAPTER FOURTEEN 66

CHAPTER SIXTEEN 72

CHAPTER SEVENTEEN 77

Successful Gamification Approaches. 77

CHAPTER EIGHTEEN 81

CHAPTER NINTEEN 84

The Importance of Understanding the Importance of Employee Assistance Programs. 84

CHAPTER TWENTY 91

INTRODUCTION

In the modern workplace, the concept of self-care has transcended its conventional boundaries and become an indispensable part of corporate culture. As organizations increasingly recognize the intrinsic link between employee well-being and productivity, promoting *mental health* and self-care among colleagues and employees is gaining momentum. It is no longer an afterthought, but a priority in promoting a healthy, vibrant and supportive work environment. By tackling the complex terrain of *mental health care, we empower individuals to manage stress, build resilience and thrive professionally and personally.*

Let's delve into this crucial facet of the broader discussion about addressing *mental health* issues in the workplace:

CHAPTER ONE

Redefine self-care:

Self-care is often misinterpreted as simply a day at the spa or a relaxing walk in the park. While these are valid forms of self-care, it goes far beyond pampering. It is essential that colleagues and employees are encouraged to view self-care as a holistic concept that encompasses physical, emotional and psychological well-being. For example, it might mean encouraging regular breaks during the workday, practicing mindfulness, or setting clear boundaries between work and home life. By redefining self-care, we empower individuals to proactively take control of their *mental health*.

Creating **a supportive environment:**

The workplace itself plays a crucial role in promoting self-care. Encourage open conversations about mental health and destigmatize seeking help. For example, having designated mental health resources or Employee Assistance Programs (EAPs) can be invaluable. Additionally, offering flexibility in work arrangements, such as remote work or flexible hours, can help employees better balance their professional and personal lives, reducing stress and burnout.

Encourage physical well-being:

A healthy body often translates into a healthy mind. Promote physical activities and good nutrition in the workplace. Simple initiatives like a standing desk, yoga classes or gym membership can make a big difference. Additionally, organizations can consider offering *mental health care days in addition to sick leave, so that employees can look after their mental wellbeing* without feeling pressured to pretend to be physically unwell.

Mental health awareness programs:

Conduct workshops or training sessions to raise awareness about mental health. Invite mental health professionals to provide insights and tools for dealing with stress, anxiety, and other common issues. Regularly scheduled seminars or webinars can ensure that information is accessible to all employees.

Lead by example:

Leaders and managers must set the tone for self-care within the organization. When they prioritize self-care and *mental health, a clear message* is sent to their teams that these aspects are important. *An example of this* could be a manager sharing his own self-care routines or openly discussing his struggles and coping strategies.

Monitor workload and expectations:

Assess the workload and expectations placed on employees. Unrealistic deadlines and overloaded schedules can significantly contribute to stress. Use performance metrics that consider both productivity and well-being, and be prepared to make adjustments as necessary.

Flexible leave:

Encourage the use of vacation days and personal leave. Some organizations even offer ' *mental health* days ' to explicitly recognize the importance of taking a break for *mental wellbeing*.

Feedback and Improvement:

Create feedback channels where employees can express their concerns, suggestions and experiences regarding self-care initiatives. Evaluate these programs regularly and adjust them based on feedback received.

peer support networks :

Promote the formation of peer support groups within the organization. Coworkers who share similar experiences can provide *valuable emotional support* and a sense of connection.

Celebrate achievements:

Recognize and celebrate milestones in self-care. Recognize individuals who have made positive changes to their self-care routines or achieved better *mental well-being*.

In this era of increased attention to mental health, encouraging self-care in the workplace is not just an HR strategy; it is a strategic business imperative. By fostering a culture that values and prioritizes mental wellbeing, organizations can unleash the full potential of their employees, leading to greater job satisfaction, *higher productivity* and reduced employee turnover. It's a win-win scenario for both employees and employers, fostering a work environment that is not only productive, but truly supportive.

CHAPTER TWO

Communicating the Value of EACAs to Employees.

One of the challenges companies face when implementing employee assistance and counseling programs (EACAs) is communicating the value of these programs to employees. Although EACAs are designed to support employee well-being, employees sometimes don't fully understand what these programs offer or they may feel hesitant to use them. It is important for companies to effectively communicate the value of EACAs to encourage employee participation and use.

From an employee perspective, there may be a stigma associated with seeking mental health support. Employees may feel judged or fear *negative consequences* for seeking help. Additionally, employees may be unaware of *the resources available* and how to have access to them. From the employer's perspective, EACAs can be seen as *an additional cost* and cannot be prioritized over other company initiatives.

To address these challenges, here are *some ways* to effectively communicate the value of EACAs to employees:

1. **Provide clear and concise information:** Ensure employees have access to information about the resources available. This includes the types of services offered, how to access them and any associated costs. Providing this information in a clear and concise manner will help employees help them understand what is available to them and how to get help when they need it.

2. **Address the stigma associated with mental health**: Companies can work to reduce the stigma associated with seeking mental health care by normalizing the conversation around mental health. This can be done through training programs, employee resources and communication campaigns that promote mental health awareness.

3. **Highlight the benefits of EACAS**: It is important to communicate the benefits of EACAs to employees. This includes the impact on employee well-being, improved work performance and reduced absenteeism. Providing real-life examples of how EACAS has helped employees can also be effective in highlighting the value of these programs.

4. **Encourage leadership support:** When leaders are open about their own experiences with mental health and the benefits of EACAS, it can help reduce the stigma associated

with seeking support. Encouraging leadership to promote the use of EACAs. can also help to increase employee participation.

By effectively communicating the value of EACAs to employees, companies can encourage participation and use of these programs. This can ultimately lead to *improved* employee well-being and job performance.

CHAPTER THREE

Understanding **the Importance of Mental Health in Childcare Professionals:**

- **Nuance**: Working in childcare can be both rewarding and demanding. Childcare professionals often face high levels of stress due to long working hours, emotional labor and the responsibility of caring for *young children*.

- **Perspective 1**: From a child care worker's perspective, maintaining good *mental health* is essential to providing quality care. Burnout, compassion fatigue, and *vicarious trauma* are common challenges.

- **Perspective 2**: Employers and policy makers recognize that a mentally healthy workforce is crucial to *the overall well-being* of children. When caregivers are mentally healthy, they can create *a positive environment* for children's growth.

- **Example**: *A childcare worker named* Maria shares her experience of feeling overwhelmed by the demands of her job. She emphasizes the need for self-care and emotional support.

Strategies to support mental health and well-being:

- **Nuance**: *Effective strategies* can reduce stress and promote the well-being of childcare professionals.

- **Perspective 1: Self-care practices**:

- Encourage employees to prioritize self-care. This includes *regular breaks*, exercise and mindfulness.

- *Provide resources such as counseling services or stress management workshops.*

- Example: The children's center offers *weekly yoga sessions* for employees.

- **Perspective 2: Workplace policies and support**:

- Implement policies that address work-life balance, workload and *fair pay*.

- Create *a supportive work environment* in which colleagues and managers actively listen and empathize.

- Example: The center allows flexible working hours and offers *mental health* care days.

- **Perspective 3: Training and education**:

- Train staff to recognize signs of burnout and stress in themselves and their colleagues.

- Teach them about coping strategies and techniques for building resilience.

- Example: The annual professional development conference includes sessions on mental health awareness.

- **Perspective 4** : **Community and peer support** :

- *Promoting a sense of community* among childcare workers.

- Encourage peer support groups or mentorship programs.

- Example: The center organizes *monthly meetings* where employees share experiences and coping strategies.

3. **Challenges and Considerations**:

- **Nuance**: Despite efforts, challenges remain.

- **Perspective 1**: *Stigma and silence*:

- Some employees are hesitant to seek help due to the stigma surrounding *mental health*.

- Normalize conversations about *mental well-being*.

- Example: Center leadership openly discusses their own mental health journey.

- **Perspective 2**: **Resource constraints**:

- Many centers operate on tight budgets, limiting access to mental health care.

- Advocate for increased funding and resource allocation.

- Example: A local nonprofit organization partners with child care centers to offer *free counseling sessions*.

4. **Conclusion**:

- **Nuance**: prioritizing *mental health* in childcare benefits everyone involved: the professionals, the children and the families.

- **Perspective**: Let's recognize the resilience of childcare workers and actively support their well-being. By doing this we create *a nurturing environment* in which children thrive.

Remember that the well-being of childcare professionals directly affects the quality of care they provide. Let's continue to advocate for expanded mental health support in the child care sector.

CHAPTER FOUR

The Intersection of Outcome Regret and Mental Health.

Result regret is a complex emotional experience that can have a significant impact on mental health. When individuals experience regret about the outcome of their decisions, it can lead to feelings of sadness, anxiety, and even depression. This is especially true if the regret is related to a major decision, such as a career choice or a major life event. The intersection of outcome regret and *mental health* is an area of research that has received increasing attention in recent years.

1. Research has shown that regret about the outcome can have a negative effect on *mental health*. A study conducted by JA Stein et al. (2012) found that individuals who regretted a major life decision were more likely to report symptoms of depression

and anxiety. This suggests that regret about the outcome may contribute to the development of *mental disorders*.

2. Regret about the outcome can also be a symptom of mental disorders. For example, people with depression may experience regret about their past decisions or actions. This can be the result of negative self-talk and a focus on past mistakes. Likewise, people with anxiety may experience regret related to their decisions due to worry and fear of making the wrong choice.

3. The relationship between outcome regret and *mental health* is complex and bidirectional. While regret about the outcome can contribute to the development of *mental disorders*, *mental disorders* can also contribute to the experience of regret about the outcome. For example, people with low self-esteem or *negative self-image* are more likely to regret their decisions because they tend to focus on their mistakes.

4. Treating mental disorders can help individuals manage outcome regret. Cognitive behavioral therapy (CBT) is a form of therapy that can be particularly effective in treating outcome regret. CBT focuses on changing *negative thought patterns* and behaviors, which can help individuals, develop a more positive view of their decisions and reduce *feelings of regret*.

5. It is important to note that not all regrets are negative. Regret can also be a positive emotion that motivates people to make *positive changes* in their lives. For example, regret over a career choice can motivate someone to pursue a different career path that is more fulfilling.

The intersection of outcome regret and *mental health* is a complex area of research that requires further research. While regret about the outcome can have a negative impact on *mental health*, it is important to recognize that not all regret is negative and it can also be a positive motivator for change. Understand emphasizes personalized care for individuals with complex health problems, including mental disorders. ICCH brings together various healthcare providers, including mental health specialists, to provide *coordinated care* that addresses all aspects of a patient's health. This approach is aimed at improving patient outcomes and reducing healthcare costs.

2. How can ICCH help with mental health treatment?

ICCH can aid *mental health* treatment in several ways. First, ICCH provides *personalized care* that meets the unique needs of each patient. Mental health disorders are complex and can have *several underlying causes*, including genetics, environment, and lifestyle factors. ICCH considers all of these factors in developing a treatment plan, which can lead to *better outcomes* for patients.

Second, ICCH provides coordinated care across multiple healthcare providers. Mental health disorders often require multiple types of treatment, including medications, therapy, and lifestyle changes. ICCH ensures that all of these treatments work together to achieve the best possible outcomes for patients.

3. What are the challenges of implementing ICCH for *mental health* treatment?

Implementing ICCH for *mental health* treatment can be challenging. One of the key challenges is the lack of coordination among different healthcare providers. Mental health treatment often involves multiple providers, including primary care physicians, psychiatrists, and therapists. These providers may communicate do not interact effectively with each other, leading to *fragmented care*.

Another challenge is the lack of resources for *mental health* treatment. Mental health services are often underfunded, leading to long wait times and limited access to care. ICCH requires *additional resources* to implement effectively, which can be difficult to obtain.

4. *What are some examples of ICCH in mental health* treatment ?

There are several examples of ICCH in mental health treatment. One example is the collaborative care model, which involves a team of healthcare providers working together to provide *coordinated care* to patients with depression. This model has been shown to improve patient outcomes improves and reduces healthcare costs.

Another example is the stepped care model, in which the least intensive treatment is provided first and the level of care is increased as needed. This model is particularly useful for patients with mild to moderate *mental disorders.*

5. *What is the best option for ICCH in mental health* treatment?

The best option for ICCH in mental health treatment depends on the specific needs of each patient. However, a combination of the collaborative care model and the stepped care model may be the most effective approach. This approach provides *personalized care* that meets the unique needs of every patient, while also ensuring that all providers work together to provide *coordinated care. Additionally,* the stepped care model ensures that patients receive *the least invasive treatment* first, which can reduce the risk of side effects and improve outcomes.

ICCH is a promising approach to *personalized mental health* treatment. It provides coordinated care across healthcare providers and considers all aspects of a patient's health. While there are challenges to implementing ICCH for *mental health treatment, several successful* approaches exist models. A combination of *the collaborative care model* and the step-by-step care model can be the most effective approach.

CHAPTER FIVE

Fundraising Strategies for Mental Health Care.

Fundraising strategies for mental health issues

In our quest to support mental health awareness and advocate for those affected by mental illness, *effective fundraising strategies* play a crucial role. These strategies not only raise much-needed funds, but also promote community involvement, spread awareness, and create *lasting impact.* Let's explore different approaches from different perspectives:

1. **Community Events and Campaigns:**

- **Walkathons and *Fun Runs*:** Organizing community walks, running or cycling events can bring people together and raise *money at the same time.* Participants can seek sponsorship from friends, family and colleagues.

Case in point: The "Mindful Miles" walkathon raised $50,000 for a local *mental health* clinic last year.

- **Art exhibitions and concerts:** collaborate with *local artists*, musicians and performers to organize events. Ticket sales, art auctions and merchandise revenues can contribute to this.

Example: The 'Healing through Art' exhibition featured artwork with *a mental health theme* and raised awareness.

- **Social media challenges:** Create viral challenges (like the ALS Ice Bucket Challenge) related to *mental health*. *Encourage participants* to donate and nominate others.

Example: The #Mindful Elfie challenge raised money for mental *health* research.

2. Corporate Partnerships:

- **Employee Giving Programs:** Work with companies to set up payroll deductions or matching gift programs. Employees can donate part of their salary and the company will match the contribution.

Example: XYZ Corporation doubled employee donations to a mental health nonprofit during *Mental Health Awareness* Month.

- **Charity Marketing Campaigns:** Work with companies to create charity-related marketing campaigns. A percentage of sales from specific products or services can go to *mental health* initiatives.

Example: A popular coffee chain donated $1 from every 'Mindful Brew' sold to *mental health* organizations.

3. **Online Fundraising Platforms:**

- **Crowd funding:** use platforms such as GoFundMe, Kickstarter or Indiegogo to create campaigns. Share compelling stories and progress updates to engage donors.

Example: *A young woman* received therapy for her anxiety disorder through a crowdfunding campaign.

- **Peer-to-peer fundraising:** Encourage supporters to create their own fundraising pages. They can ask friends and family to make a donation on their behalf.

Example: John's birthday fundraiser raised $1,000 for suicide prevention.

4. **Grant applications and foundations:**

- **Research grants:** apply for grants from research foundations in the field of *mental health*. These funds support studies, *clinical trials* and *innovative treatments*.

Example: The 'Hope for Tomorrow' foundation awarded a $100,000 grant to study mindfulness-based interventions.

- **Community Grants: Local government agencies and private foundations often offer grants for** *mental health* programs. Create compelling proposals that highlight the impact of your initiative.

Example: The Community Wellness Grant funded a series of *mental health* workshops for youth.

5. *Legacy Gifts* **and Donations:**

- **Planned Giving:** Encourage supporters to include your organization in their wills or estate plans. Be transparent about how these gifts will benefit *mental health* goals.

Example: Longtime advocate Jane left a generous donation to establish a *mental health scholarship*.

- **Endowment Funds**: Create an endowment fund that keeps the principal intact and uses only investment income. This ensures *sustainable financing*.

Example: The 'Mindful Futures' donation annually supports mental health education programs.

Remember, successful fundraising isn't just about dollars raised; it's about building a compassionate community behind *mental health* causes. Every contribution, big or small, contributes to *a brighter, more empathetic world*.

Feel free to adapt and expand these strategies based on *your specific context* and target group. Together we can make a difference!

CHAPTER SIX

General well-being first.

1. **Awareness and education:**

- **Employee training programs**: Organizations should invest in regular training sessions that raise awareness about mental health issues. These programs can cover topics such as stress management, emotional intelligence, and recognizing signs of burnout.

- **Stigma reduction**: Encourage open conversations about mental health. By reducing the stigma associated with seeking help, employees are more likely to reach out when they need support.

2. *Flexible working arrangements*:

- **Remote working**: The pandemic has highlighted the importance of flexible working arrangements. Allowing employees to work remotely or offering *flexible hours can significantly reduce stress levels.*

- **Compressed workweeks**: Some companies are experimenting with *shorter workweeks (for example, four 10-hour* days) to give employees more time for self-care and family.

3. **Relationship between physical health and mental health:**

- **Exercise**: regular physical activity has a positive impact on *mental health. Encourage employees* to take breaks for *a short walk* or participate in fitness challenges.

- **Nutrition**: a balanced diet influences mood and cognitive function. Consider, for example, offering *healthy snacks* or organizing nutrition workshops.

4. **Work-Life Balance:**

- **Setting boundaries**: Encourage employees to set clear boundaries between work and private life. Avoiding emails outside of office hours and respecting weekends can prevent burnout.

- **Vacation policy**: ensure that employees take their vacation days. A break from work rejuvenates the mind and prevents *chronic stress*.

5. *Supportive leadership*:

- **Lead by example**: Managers should **prioritize their own mental health** and demonstrate self-care practices. This sets *a positive tone* for *the entire team*.

- **Empathy and compassion**: Leaders who *actively listen* and demonstrate empathy create *a psychologically safe environment*. Employees feel comfortable discussing their challenges.

6. **Access to Resources:**

- **Employee Assistance Programs (EAPs)** : EAPs provide confidential counseling services to employees. Make sure employees know how to access these resources.

- *Mental Health* **Days**: Consider allowing specific days off for *mental health* reasons. Recognize that *mental health* is just as important as *physical health*.

7. Promoting work-life integration:

- **Flexible schedules**: Allow employees to attend family events or personal obligations during work hours. Trust them to manage their time effectively.

- **Parental Leave**: Expand parental leave policies to support *new parents during critical life transitions*.

Examples:

- *Company X* implemented a 'Wellness Wednesday' initiative where employees participate in mindfulness sessions during lunch breaks.

- *Tech Startup Y offers unlimited paid leave for mental health* reasons, emphasizing the importance of self-care.

- *Healthcare provider Z offers free counseling sessions* for employees and their families through their EAP.

Keep in mind that prioritizing *mental wellness* is not just a trend, but a vital investment in the long-term health and productivity of your workforce. By promoting *a mentally healthy workplace, organizations can create a positive ripple effect* that extends beyond the office walls.

I have provided an extensive section on prioritizing *mental wellbeing*, including insights from different perspectives and using examples to illustrate key points. If you need more details or *additional content, please ask!*

CHAPTER SEVEN

The link between emotional well-being and mental disorders.

Emotions are an inherent part of the human experience and shape our thoughts, actions and our overall well-being. Although emotions can be both positive and negative, they play a crucial role in our mental health. The way we process and regulate our emotions can have a profound impact on our psychological well-being, and conversely, mental health issues can significantly impact our emotional state. In this section, we explore the complicated link between *emotional well-being* and mental health disorders, shedding light on the ways in which our emotions can influence our *mental health*.

1. **The impact of unresolved emotions on *mental health*:**

Unresolved emotions, such as sadness, anger or trauma, can have a lasting impact on our mental health. When we suppress or ignore these emotions, they can fester and manifest as *mental disorders*. For example, someone who has experienced a traumatic event but refuses to deal with *the associated emotions* may develop post-traumatic stress disorder (PTSD). Likewise, unexpressed anger or sadness can lead to depression or anxiety disorders. It is essential to acknowledge and process our emotions in a healthy way to prevent them from negatively impacting *our mental well-being*.

2. **The role of *emotional regulation* in *mental health*:**

Emotional regulation refers to the ability to manage and control our emotions appropriately. Individuals with poor emotional regulation skills are more prone to developing mental disorders. For example, someone who has difficulty regulating their anger may be at greater risk of developing intermittent explosive disorder. On the other hand, individuals who have effective **emotional regulation skills** are better equipped to manage stress, maintain healthy relationships, and prevent the onset of mental health problems. Developing *emotional regulation* techniques, such as mindfulness or therapy, can be helpful in promoting *overall mental well-being*.

3. The influence of mental health on *emotional well-being*:

Just as emotions can impact *mental health*, mental disorders can significantly impact our emotional well-being. Conditions such as depression, anxiety or bipolar disorder can distort our perception of reality and disrupt our emotional balance. For example, people with depression may experience a persistent feeling of sadness or hopelessness, making it challenging for them to experience positive emotions. Understanding the interplay between *mental health* and emotions is crucial to providing effective treatment and support for people with *mental health disorders*.

4. The Importance of Seeking Help:

Recognizing the connection between emotions and mental health underlines the importance of seeking professional help when needed. Mental health professionals, such as therapists or psychiatrists, can provide guidance and support in navigating the complex relationship between emotions and mental disorders. Additionally, therapy can help individuals develop healthy coping mechanisms, improve emotional regulation skills, and address unresolved emotions. Remember that seeking help is not a sign of weakness, but rather a proactive step toward nurturing *our emotional and mental well-being.*

Emotions and mental health are closely linked, influencing each other in profound ways. Understanding and addressing the link between emotional well-being and mental health disorders is critical in promoting overall mental well-being. By acknowledging and processing our emotions, developing effective emotional regulation skills, and seeking professional help when needed, we can strive to achieve *a healthier and more balanced state of mind.*

CHAPTER EIGHT

How Mental Health Startups Are Changing Lives: Overcoming Challenges: Regulation and Ethics in Mental Health Startups.

1. Understanding the *regulatory landscape*

One of the **biggest challenges** *mental health* startups face is navigating the complex and ever-changing regulatory landscape. The field of *mental health* is highly regulated and for good reason. Patients' well-being and safety are at stake, making it imperative for startups in this space to ensure compliance with *all relevant regulations*.

For example, a mental health startup that develops a mobile app to provide therapy services must comply with privacy laws, such as the Portability and Accountability Act (HIPAA) in the

United States. This means implementing secure systems to protect patient data and obtain *necessary consent* from users.

2. Balancing innovation with *ethical considerations*

While mental health startups strive to innovate and develop new technologies and approaches to improve mental health care, they must also carefully consider *the ethical implications* of their work. It is essential to strike a balance between pushing boundaries and ensuring patient safety and well-being.

For example, a startup that offers virtual reality therapy must consider ethical concerns regarding the potential risks and side effects of immersive experiences. They must conduct thorough research and testing to ensure that their technology is safe and effective, and that it does not harm those who use it.

3. Build trust and credibility

Establishing trust and credibility is crucial for *mental health* startups, especially in an industry where patients' lives are directly affected. Overcoming skepticism and gaining the trust of both patients and healthcare professionals can be a key challenge.

To overcome this, startups must demonstrate transparency and accountability. They must clearly communicate their mission, values, and approach to *mental health care. Additionally,* startups can build credibility by partnering with established *mental health* organizations, collaborating with renowned clinicians, and rigorous conduct *clinical trials to validate the effectiveness of their products or services.*

4. Collaborate with regulators and industry experts

To navigate the regulatory challenges and ensure ethical practices, mental health startups must actively collaborate with regulators and industry experts. By engaging in open dialogue and seeking guidance from relevant authorities, startups can help stay informed staying up to date with the latest regulations and *best practices*.

For example, startups can participate in industry associations and conferences, where they can network with regulators and experts in the field. By proactively engaging with the regulatory community, startups can gain insight into *upcoming changes* and help shape regulations that are fair, effective and support innovation.

5. Embrace ethical design principles

Ethical design principles should be at the core of any mental health startup's product or service. Designing with empathy and considering the potential impact on *vulnerable populations* is essential.

For example, a mental health app should prioritize users' privacy and data protection; ensuring *personal information* is stored securely and used only for its intended purpose. The app should also provide clear instructions and resources for seeking *professional help* when is needed, rather than relying solely on *digital interventions*.

By incorporating ethical design principles, startups can not only meet regulatory requirements, but also build trust and promote positive user experiences, ultimately contributing to the overall success and impact of their ventures.

In conclusion, mental health startups face significant challenges when it comes to regulation and ethics. By understanding the regulatory landscape, balancing innovation with ethical considerations, building trust and credibility, collaborating with regulators and industry experts industry and ethical design principles, startups can overcome these challenges and positively impact *mental health care*.

CHAPTER NINE

Sharing personal experiences on a mental health blog.

1. Stories have always played an important role in human communication and understanding. They have the power to transport us to different worlds, evoke emotions and create connections between individuals. But did you know that storytelling is also a powerful tool can be for healing and promoting mental wellness? In recent years, blogs in the *mental health* field have emerged as safe spaces for individuals to share their *personal experiences* and journeys and provide a source of support, validation and inspiration to others who may be going through *similar struggles*.

2. When individuals bravely share their personal experiences on a mental health blog, they create a sense of community and understanding. This act of vulnerability not only allows the writer to process their own emotions, but also provides comfort to readers who may feel alone in their own battles. For example, a blog post about overcoming anxiety might describe the writer's journey, including the challenges they faced, the coping mechanisms they discovered, and the progress they made. Through their story, the writer not only feels a sense of relief, but also offers hope and encouragement to others who are still struggling with fear.

3. Additionally, storytelling on **mental health** blogs helps break down stigmas surrounding *mental health*. *When individuals openly discuss their struggles and triumphs, they contribute to the normalization of mental health* issues in society. A blog post about living with depression, for example, can explore the writer's daily experiences, such as the impact of depression on their relationships, work, and *general well-being*. By shedding light on

these topics, the writer helps to educate others and dispel misconceptions about *mental illness*.

4. Additionally, sharing personal experiences on a mental health blog can be a cathartic and therapeutic process for the writer. Self-writing can serve as a form of self-expression and self-reflection, allowing individuals to better understand their own emotions and experiences. Through the process of creating a blog post, writers can discover new insights, gain clarity, and find a sense of release from their struggles. In turn, this can lead to personal growth and *a deeper connection* with themselves.

5. Finally, the power of storytelling lies in its ability to inspire and motivate others. When individuals share their personal stories of resilience and recovery, they provide a beacon of hope to those who may feel hopeless or defeated. These stories can serve as reminders that healing is possible and that there is light at the end of the tunnel. For example, *a mental health* blog post detailing a writer's journey to self-acceptance and self-love

can provide *invaluable inspiration* to readers who may struggle with their own self-esteem.

Through stories on *mental health* blogs, individuals can find comfort, support and empowerment. By sharing personal experiences, they contribute to a sense of community, break down stigmas and inspire others on their own journeys to mental wellness. So if you have a story to tell, consider sharing it on a *mental health* care blog, your words can have *a profound impact* on someone's life.

CHAPTER TEN

Addressing mental health in residential care.

In the healthcare field, the provision of inpatient care plays a crucial role in treating acute illnesses, managing chronic conditions, and facilitating recovery. However, amid the hustle and bustle of medical interventions, we often overlook a crucial aspect: *mental health*. The body and mind are intimately connected, and addressing mental wellness within the context of *inpatient care* is not only humane, but also *essential to holistic healing*.

Let's delve into the nuances of addressing *mental health* in *the inpatient setting*, drawing insights from several perspectives:

1. **Screening and assessment**:

- **Nuance**: Identifying *mental health* issues early is critical. *Inpatient facilities* should include *systematic screening processes* to assess *the psychological well-being of patients upon admission.*

- **Example**: A cardiac patient admitted for surgery may experience anxiety related to the procedure. *A brief anxiety assessment* can guide tailored interventions.

2. *Integrated Care Teams*:

- **Nuance**: Collaboration among healthcare professionals is critical. In *inpatient care* teams, psychiatrists, psychologists, *social workers* and nurses must work together seamlessly.

- **Example** : a patient with diabetes may suffer from depression. The endocrinologist, nurse, and psychologist work together to address both *physical and emotional needs.*

3. **Environment and safety**:

- **Nuance**: the physical environment influences *mental health*. Hospital wards should be designed to minimize stressors and promote comfort.

- **Example**: Soft lighting, *soothing colors* and private spaces contribute to *a calming atmosphere*, reducing patient anxiety.

4. *Therapeutic interventions*:

- **Nuance**: Evidence-based therapies improve mental well-being. Cognitive behavioral therapy (CBT), mindfulness and *expressive arts* can be integrated.

- **Example**: A cancer patient coping with pain may benefit from CBT sessions to manage pain and improve pain tolerance.

5. **Family Involvement**:

- **Nuance**: Families are *an integral part* of the healing process. Inpatient care must actively involve family members in treatment planning.

- **Example**: A child admitted for an asthma exacerbation thrives when parents participate in asthma education and *emotional support*.

6. **Stigma Reduction**:

- **Nuance**: Mental health stigma persists. *Inpatient settings* must create an environment where patients feel safe to discuss *their emotional problems.*

- **Example**: A young adult with *bipolar disorder* should feel comfortable sharing symptoms without fear of judgment.

7. **Transition planning**:

- **Nuance**: Preparing patients for discharge is critical. Addressing *mental health* during this phase ensures continuity of care.

- **Example**: *A postoperative patient* receives *a personalized care plan* that includes follow-up appointments with a psychiatrist.

8. **Staff training and support**:

- **Nuance**: Healthcare providers need training in mental health awareness. *Supportive supervision* and debriefing sessions are essential.

- **Example**: Nurses learn de-escalation techniques to deal with *agitated patients, promoting safety and trust.*

9. **Patient Empowerment:**

- **Nuance**: inpatient care should enable patients to actively participate in their *mental health* care.

- **Example:** A stroke survivor attends group therapy sessions, shares experiences, and learns coping strategies from peers.

10. *Holistic Statistics*:

- **Nuance**: in addition to physical parameters, the results of inpatient care should also include *mental health* indicators.

- **Example:** Tracking anxiety levels sleep quality and *emotional distress* provides *a comprehensive view* of patient progress.

Revolutionizing inpatient care necessitates that *mental health* be recognized as an integral part of the healing journey.

By addressing *mental wellbeing with sensitivity, empathy and evidence-based practices, we can make a real difference in patients' lives.*

CHAPTER ELEVEN

Inspiring Stories of Industry Triumph: Giving Back: Entrepreneurs Making a Difference in Health and Wellness .

1. Provide access to *affordable healthcare*

One way entrepreneurs in the health and wellness industry are making a difference is by focusing on providing access to *affordable healthcare*. They understand that not everyone has the means to pay for *expensive medical treatments* or consultations, and they do everything they can to bridge this gap.

For example, entrepreneur Jane Smith has founded a telehealth platform that connects patients with doctors who offer *affordable consultations online*. Through this platform, individuals can receive *medical advice* and prescriptions without the burden of *high costs* or *long wait times*. By making healthcare more accessible and affordable, Jane helps people take back control of their health and well-being.

2. Promoting mental health awareness

In recent years, there has been increasing recognition of the importance of mental health. Entrepreneurs in the health and wellbeing sector play a crucial role in promoting *mental health* awareness and providing support to people struggling with *mental health* issues.

Take the example of John Doe, who started a *mental health* care app that provides resources, self-help, and a supportive community for people dealing with anxiety and depression. Through his app, John not only helps people find comfort and support, but also reduces the stigma surrounding *mental health*. By using technology to reach a wide audience, he has *a significant impact* on people's lives.

3. Empowering individuals through fitness education

Other way entrepreneurs are making a difference in health and wellness is by empowering individuals through fitness education. They understand that knowledge is power, and by equipping people with *the right information* they can make informed decisions about their health and well-being.

For example, Sarah Johnson, a fitness entrepreneur, offers online courses and workshops that teach people about good nutrition, exercise techniques, and overall wellness. Through her educational programs, Sarah empowers people to take control of their physical health and make *positive changes* to their lifestyle. By providing *valuable knowledge* and guidance, she helps individuals achieve their fitness goals and live healthier lives.

4. Support sustainable and ethical practices

Entrepreneurs in the health and wellness sector are also making a difference by adopting sustainable and ethical practices. They recognize the impact their businesses can have on the environment and take steps to minimize their carbon footprint.

For example, Mike Thompson, the founder of a sustainable skin care brand, sources ingredients from organic farms and uses eco-friendly packaging materials. By prioritizing sustainability and *ethical sourcing*, Mike not only creates products that benefit consumers, but also preserve the planet for *future generations*.

Conclusion:

These are just a few examples of how health and wellness entrepreneurs are giving back and making a significant difference in people's lives. Whether it's providing affordable healthcare, promoting *mental health* awareness, offering fitness education, or adopting *sustainable practices*, these entrepreneurs are using their platforms to make a positive impact. Their efforts are not only inspiring, but a reminder of the power of entrepreneurship in creating a healthier and happier world.

Entrepreneurs are misfits to the core. They forge ahead, making their own path and always, always, question the status quo.
Maximillian DeGeneres

CHAPTER TWELVE

Creating Authentic and Compassionate Messages .

Creating authentic and compassionate messages is a crucial aspect of supporting mental health goals and raising awareness. It's about creating messages that resonate with individuals, convey empathy and promote understanding. By using authentic and *compassionate messaging,* organizations can *effectively* connect with their audiences and create *positive change*.

When developing authentic and compassionate messages, it is important to consider different perspectives. This provides a comprehensive understanding of the diverse experiences and challenges that individuals face with *mental health issues*. By integrating insights from different points of view, organizations can create messages that are inclusive, relatable and respectful.

To provide in-depth information on this topic, I will present a numbered list of key considerations for creating authentic and *compassionate messages*:

1. Empathy: Authentic messaging requires a deep sense of empathy. It is essential to understand the emotions and struggles that people with mental health problems may face. By acknowledging their experiences and showing empathy, organizations can build trust and create a supportive environment.

2. Language and tone: The choice of language and tone plays an important role in conveying compassion. Using non-stigmatizing and non-judgmental language helps reduce the stigma surrounding *mental health* . It's important to strike a balance between being informative and sensitive, while ensuring the message is respectful and supportive.

3. Personal Stories: Sharing personal stories can be a powerful way to create *authentic messages*. By showcasing real-life experiences from individuals who have overcome *mental health* challenges or are still on their way, organizations can inspire hope and provide *relatable examples* for their audiences.

4. Education and Awareness: Authentic messaging should also focus on educating and raising awareness about mental health. Providing accurate information, dispelling myths and promoting understanding can help reduce stigma and encourage *open conversations.*

5. Collaboration: Collaborating with *mental health* professionals, advocates and individuals with *lived experiences* can increase the authenticity of reporting. By involving these stakeholders in the development process, organizations can ensure that *their message aligns* with the needs and perspectives of the community they seek to support.

6. Sensitivity to Triggers: It is critical to consider potential triggers when crafting *mental health* messaging . Sensitivity to

topics such as self-harm, suicide or trauma is essential to avoid causing harm or distress to those who encounter the messages.

Remember, these are general insights into creating authentic and compassionate messages for *mental health* goals. It is always recommended to consult experts and conduct *thorough research* to tailor the message to *specific contexts* and audiences.

CHAPTER THIRETEEN

Research on the impact of behavioral health education.

1. Understanding the Foundations of Behavioral Health Education:

- **Definition and scope**: Behavioral health education covers a wide range of knowledge and skills related to *mental health*, *emotional well-being* and behavioral patterns. It extends beyond *the clinical setting* to include community programs, schools, workplaces, and public health initiatives.

- **Holistic approach**: Behavioral health education recognizes that *mental health* is linked to *physical health*, *social factors* and environmental influences. It emphasizes *a holistic understanding* of well-being, taking into account biological, psychological and social determinants.

- **Promoting awareness**: Education in this area aims to increase awareness of *mental health* issues, reduce stigma and encourage early intervention. By disseminating *accurate information*, we empower individuals to recognize signs of distress and seek help quickly.

2. **Impact on individuals and communities:**

- **Empowering individuals**: Behavioral health education equips individuals with coping strategies, stress management techniques, and emotional resilience. When people understand their own mental health needs, they can make informed decisions and advocate for themselves.

- **Preventing mental disorders** : education plays a preventive role by promoting *healthy behavior*, stress reduction and self-care. For example:

- **Mindfulness exercises**: Learning mindfulness meditation or relaxation techniques can improve *emotional regulation* and reduce anxiety.

- **Substance abuse prevention**: Educational programs on substance abuse increase awareness of the risks and provide coping skills to prevent addiction.

- **Community Resilience**: A well-informed community is better equipped to deal with crises, whether natural disasters, pandemics or social unrest. *Behavioral health education* promotes community resilience by strengthening *social support networks* and promoting *adaptive coping mechanisms*.

3. **Integration between institutions:**

- **Schools and universities**: Incorporating behavioral health education into curricula helps students develop **skills in emotional intelligence**, empathy and conflict resolution. It's also about bullying, peer pressure and *academic stress*.

- **Workplaces**: Employee wellness programs often include mental health components. Training managers and colleagues to recognize signs of anxiety can create a supportive work environment.

- **Primary Care Clinics**: Integrating behavioral health education into routine medical visits ensures patients understand the relationship between the mind and body. In addition to physical health, doctors can also talk about stress management, sleep hygiene, and *emotional well-being* .

4. *Cultural competence* **and diversity** :

- **Customizing education**: recognizing cultural differences is crucial. Behavioral health education should be culturally sensitive, taking into account the diverse beliefs, practices, and stigmas associated with *mental health*.

- **Addressing disparities**: By understanding cultural nuances, educators can bridge gaps in access to mental health care. For example:

- **Language barriers**: offering *educational material* in multiple languages ensures *a greater reach*.

- **Stigma reduction**: culturally *competent education* challenges stereotypes and encourages *open dialogue*.

5. **Practical examples**:

- **Peer-Led Support Groups**: Peer educators who have experienced *mental health* issues themselves lead support groups. These groups provide *a safe space* for sharing experiences and coping strategies.

- **Online platforms**: Educational websites, podcasts and social media campaigns disseminate information widely. For example, the 'It's OK to Not Be OK' campaign encourages open conversations about *mental health*.

- **Community Workshops**: Local organizations provide workshops on stress management, parenting skills and *emotional well-being*. These workshops provide participants *with practical tools*.

In summary, behavioral health education is a dynamic force that empowers individuals, strengthens communities, and contributes to overall well-being. By embracing *diverse perspectives* and integrating education across environments, we can create *a more mentally resilient society*.

CHAPTER FOURTEEN

The Role of Mental Health in Cognitive Disorders .

In the complex web of factors that contribute to cognitive disorders, mental health plays a crucial and multifaceted role. The relationship between mental well-being and cognitive functioning is dynamic, with numerous interconnected elements that can influence each other in profound ways. As we delve into this complicated interplay, we explore the perspectives of medical professionals, researchers, and individuals who have experienced cognitive disorders firsthand. This multifaceted exploration will shed light on the complex relationship between mental health and cognitive impairment in the context of Chronic Fatigue Syndrome (CFS), commonly known as Myalgic Encephalomyelitis (ME). Here are some key insights to consider:

1. Psychological stress as a precursor:

Cognitive impairment in CFS is often exacerbated by *psychological stress*. The overwhelming and persistent nature of CFS symptoms can lead to increased levels of stress and anxiety. This in turn can further impair cognitive function, creating a vicious cycle. For example, the constant uncertainty and unpredictability of CFS symptoms can lead to *chronic stress*, which affects *cognitive performance*, memory and concentration.

2. The impact of mood disorders:

Mood disorders, such as depression and anxiety, are common companions of CFS. These mental health conditions can contribute significantly to *cognitive impairment*. For example, people with depression may experience *cognitive symptoms* such as "brain fog," which makes it challenging to concentrate and process information. Additionally, the fatigue and pain associated with CFS can worsen depressive symptoms, leading to a vicious cycle of *cognitive decline*.

3. Neurotransmitter Imbalances:

CFS is believed to be associated with disruptions in the balance of neurotransmitters, such as serotonin and dopamine, which are crucial for mood regulation and cognitive function. These imbalances can manifest as *cognitive problems*, affecting memory, problem solving, and decision-making. Addressing these neurotransmitter imbalances is essential for improving *cognitive function* in CFS patients.

4. Coping strategies and resilience:

Although mental health issues can contribute to cognitive impairment in CFS, an individual's psychological resilience and coping strategies also play an important role. Those who develop effective strategies to manage stress and anxiety may experience milder *cognitive symptoms*. For example, techniques such as mindfulness meditation and *cognitive behavioral therapy* have been shown to help CFS patients manage their *mental health and subsequently improve their cognitive function.*

5. Medicines and Their Effects:

Some medications prescribed to treat CFS symptoms or comorbid mental health conditions can have a direct impact on cognitive function. For example, certain antidepressants may improve mood but cause *cognitive side effects*. Patients and caregivers must carefully weigh the pros and cons of medications to find *the right balance for each individual*.

6. The role of sleep:

Cognitive impairment is often exacerbated in CFS due to sleep disturbances. Sleep problems, such as insomnia or hypersomnia, are common in CFS patients and may be closely linked to mental health problems. For example, poor sleep quality can worsen mood disorders, which in turn affect cognitive performance. Improving sleep hygiene is essential to address this aspect of *cognitive impairment in CFS*.

7. *Social Support* and Isolation:

The social and emotional aspects of mental health also play an important role in *cognitive disorders*. CFS patients who experience social isolation and do not have a strong support system may be more vulnerable to the negative effects of *mental health* problems on *cognitive function*. Building a robust support network can help buffer some of *the cognitive challenges* associated with CFS.

8. The Power of Rehabilitation:

Rehabilitation strategies, both cognitive and physical, can be effective in alleviating cognitive impairment associated with CFS. Cognitive rehabilitation programs, which often include exercises and activities designed to boost mental function, can improve memory, concentration, and overall cognitive skills. Additionally, addressing *mental health* issues through therapy and counseling can be a crucial part of the rehabilitation process.

The relationship between mental health and *cognitive impairment* in the context of CFS is complex and multifaceted. Understanding how psychological well-being, stress, mood disorders, **neurotransmitter imbalances, coping strategies, medications, sleep, social support, and rehabilitation interact is essential when** confronting *cognitive impairment* in CFS. By addressing the aspects of mental health, individuals and healthcare professionals can take a more comprehensive approach to managing *cognitive impairment* and improving *the overall quality of life* for people living with *this challenging condition*.

CHAPTER SIXTEEN

Supporting Wellbeing in the Workplace.

In the fast-paced world of entrepreneurship, where stress and burnout often lurk, prioritizing mental health is no longer a luxury, but a necessity. Entrepreneurs, like all professionals, face unique challenges that can negatively impact their well-being. From dealing with high stakes and financial pressure to juggling multiple roles, the demands can be overwhelming. In this section, we delve into the nuances of Mental Health First Aid (MHFA) and explore how it can be *a powerful tool* to support wellness in the workplace.

1. **Understanding MHFA:**

- **What is MHFA?** MHFA is similar to traditional first aid, but for mental health. It equips individuals with the skills to recognize and respond to signs of mental health problems in others. Just as we learn CPR to save lives during cardiac emergencies, MHFA teaches us how to provide initial support to someone experiencing a *mental health* crisis.

- **Why is it relevant?** Entrepreneurs often work in high-pressure environments, where stress, anxiety and depression can manifest. MHFA helps create a compassionate work culture by promoting empathy and reducing the stigma around *mental health*.

- **Example:** Imagine an entrepreneur notices a team member's disengagement and change in behavior. Instead of brushing it off, they start a conversation, actively listen and encourage them to seek *professional help*. *This simple action* can prevent a crisis from escalating.

2. **The role of MHFA in the workplace:**

- **Early Intervention:** MHFA encourages early intervention. Just as we address physical injuries quickly, we must do the same for *mental health* issues. Entrepreneurs who are MHFA certified can recognize warning signs and provide timely support.

- Create **a supportive environment:** entrepreneurs can set a good example. By talking openly about *mental health, sharing personal experiences* and promoting self-care, they create a workplace where employees feel safe seeking help.

- **Example:** A startup founder shares his struggle with anxiety during a team meeting. This vulnerability encourages others to open up, creating a sense of community and trust.

3. **MHFA techniques:**

- **Listen actively:** entrepreneurs trained in MHFA listen actively without judgment. They validate feelings, ask *open-ended questions*, and provide *a non-threatening space* for disclosure.

- **Provide *emotional support*:** Sometimes all someone needs is a sympathetic ear. Entrepreneurs can provide *emotional support* by acknowledging feelings and expressing empathy.

- **Example:** When an employee confiding that he is feeling overwhelmed, an entrepreneur responds, "I appreciate you sharing this with me. Let's explore ways to lighten your workload."

4. **Self-care for entrepreneurs:**

- **Recognizing their own limits:** Entrepreneurs often neglect their well-being while pursuing business goals. MHFA reminds them to prioritize self-care and seek help when needed.

- **Setting boundaries:** Entrepreneurs cannot pour from an empty cup. By setting boundaries, they model *healthy behavior* for their team.

- **Example:** an entrepreneur blocks time during his workday for meditation or exercise, demonstrating that well-being is important.

In summary, MHFA is not just a certificate; it is a commitment to promoting a mentally healthy workplace. Entrepreneurs who embrace MHFA contribute to a culture where everyone's well-being is valued, and that's an investment with *immeasurable returns*.

CHAPTER SEVENTEEN

Successful Gamification Approaches.

1. *Personalized Challenges* **and Rewards:**

- **Nuance**: One of the most important aspects of *successful gamification* is personalization. Matching challenges and rewards to an individual's preferences, goals and progress is critical.

- **Example**: Imagine a *mental health* care app that encourages users to set personalized goals related to stress reduction or mindfulness. As users complete daily meditation sessions or do positive self-talk exercises, they earn *virtual badges* or unlock new features. The app adapts to their progress and offers *relevant challenges* and rewards based on *their unique journey.*

2. *Social involvement* **and support:**

- **Nuance**: social connections play a crucial role in mental health. Gamification can increase engagement by promoting a sense of community and support.

- **Example**: Consider an online platform where users share their experiences with *mental health*, coping strategies and success stories. By participating in discussions, offering encouragement, and receiving *virtual high-fives* from colleagues, users feel connected and motivated. The gamified element can include earning points for active participation or leveling up based on *positive interactions*.

3. **Progress registration and visualization:**

- **Nuance**: transparent progress tracking helps users stay motivated. Gamification can transform data into *visually appealing representations*.

- **Example**: A mood tracking app allows users to record their emotions on a daily basis. As they enter their feelings, the app generates colorful graphs that show trends over time. Users earn streaks for consistent tracking and receive *encouraging* *messages* when they reach milestones (for *example, 30 consecutive days* of mood tracking).

4. *Stories and storytelling*:

- **Nuance**: people love stories. Gamification can weave *mental health* care pathways into *compelling stories*.

- **Example:** A *mental health* game follows the adventures of a character battling fear monsters. Players complete quests (e.g. facing *social situations*, practicing *deep breathing*) and unlock chapters of the story. The story strengthens coping skills and resilience, making the learning process engaging and memorable.

5. **Behavior reinforcement and habit formation:**

- **Nuance** : Gamification uses behavioral psychology principles to reinforce *positive habits* .

- **Example** : An app encourages users to practice gratitude daily. Every time they record something they are grateful for, they earn "gratitude coins." These coins can be exchanged for virtual items (e.g. a cozy virtual fireplace) or donated to charity. Over time, users associate gratitude with *positive rewards*, reinforcing the habit.

6. Competition and cooperation:

- **Nuance**: Balancing competition and collaboration can increase engagement.

- **Example**: A mental fitness app offers friendly challenges. Users compete for the most steps, minutes of mindfulness or acts of kindness. However, the app also encourages collaboration, for example by forming teams to jointly achieve *mental health* goals. The *competitive spirit* motivates, while teamwork promotes a sense of belonging.

Remember, successful gamification isn't about flashy graphics or superficial rewards. It's about creating meaningful experiences that empower users on their *mental health* journey. These case studies illustrate how thoughtful design and empathy can transform gamified interventions into *powerful tools* for wellness.

CHAPTER EIGHTEEN

Strategies for Addressing Presenting Employee Morale.

Presenteeism is a common problem in many workplaces and can have a significant impact on employee morale. It happens when employees come to work despite being sick, tired, or otherwise unable to perform at their full potential .This can lead to *reduced productivity* , increased stress and *a negative work environment. Tackling* presenting issues and increasing employee morale is essential to *a healthy and productive workplace. There* are several strategies that employers can implement to reduce presenting address employee morale.

1. Encourage a **healthy work-life balance**: Employers should encourage employees to take time off when they need it. This may include offering flexible work arrangements, such as

working from home or adjusting working hours, to accommodate to the needs of employees. Employers can also encourage employees to take their full vacation time and provide resources such as *mental health* days to support *their overall well-being*.

2. Promoting Employee Engagement: Engaged employees are more likely to have high morale and be productive. Employers can promote employee engagement by creating a positive work culture , providing opportunities for *professional development* , and involving employees in decision-making processes. When employees feel valued and feel involved, they are more likely to feel motivated and committed to their work.

3. Provide support for mental health: Mental health issues can contribute to presenting and low morale. Employers can provide support for mental health by offering an Employee Assistance Program (EAP), providing resources for stress management and encouraging employees to seek help when needed. Employers can also create a culture that promotes

work-life balance and recognizes the importance of mental health .

4. Celebrate successes and milestones: Recognizing employee achievements and celebrating milestones can boost morale and create a positive work environment. Employers can celebrate successes by offering rewards such as bonuses or *extra time off*. They can also celebrate achievements of recognizing employees in public and involving *the entire team* in the celebration.

Addressing presentation and increasing employee morale is essential to a healthy and productive workplace. Employers can take several steps to encourage a healthy work-life balance, promote employee engagement, provide support for mental health and celebrate successes and milestones. By implementing these strategies, employers can create a positive work environment that supports the well-being and productivity of their employees.

CHAPTER NINTEEN

The Importance of Understanding the Importance of Employee Assistance Programs.

Section 1: The Need for Employee Assistance Programs

In today's fast-paced and demanding work environments, it is essential for employers to **prioritize the well-being of their employees**. The importance of employee assistance programs (EAPs) cannot be overstated. These programs are designed to support the mental health and overall well-being of employees. They provide a wide range of services aimed at addressing the various challenges and stressors that employees may face in their personal and professional lives. From a broad perspective, the need for EAPs stems from the recognition that mental health issues can have a significant impact on an individual's performance at work. The World Health Organization estimates that depression and anxiety alone cost the global economy $1 trillion per year in *lost productivity*.

Insights:

1. EAPs are an investment in employee well-being: Employers who invest in EAPs recognize that the mental health of their employees is not only a humanitarian concern, but also a business concern. When employees face personal or professional challenges, it can lead to *reduced productivity*, increased absenteeism and higher turnover rates. EAPs provide *a structured and effective way* to tackle these problems.

2. Destigmatizing Mental Health: The existence of EAPs helps destigmatize **mental health challenges** in the workplace. By openly recognizing the importance of mental health and providing *support services, employers send a strong message* that seeking help is encouraged and accepted.

3. The role of stress in the workplace: *Modern workplaces* are often characterized by *high stress levels*. Stress can lead to

burnout, which is a growing concern for employers. EAPS can help employees cope with stress through resources such as stress management workshops, offering counseling and tools to create a healthier work-life balance.

Section 2: Services Provided by Employee Assistance Programs

One of the key features of EAPs is the wide range of services they offer. These programs are not limited to addressing a single aspect of an employee's life; rather, they provide holistic support. The services include not only mental health support health, but also help with various life challenges.

Insights:

1. Counseling and therapy: EAPs typically provide *confidential counseling services* and provide employees *with a safe space* to discuss personal and work-related issues. Examples include individual therapy for managing stress, anxiety, and depression, as well as couples or family counseling to address relationship challenges.

2. Financial and Legal Assistance: Employees may face financial and legal challenges that can impact their well-being. EAPs often provide access to *financial planners* or *legal advisors* to help employees navigate these issues. Someone dealing with debt for example, may receive guidance on budgeting and debt management.

3. Work-Life Balance and Wellness Programs: EAPs focus on improving the overall quality of life for employees. They may offer wellness programs that cover topics such as nutrition, exercise and mindfulness. These programs encourage healthier lifestyles, which both can affect an employee's personal and *professional life*.

4. Crisis Intervention: EAPs are prepared to provide immediate assistance in a crisis. Whether it is a natural disaster, workplace incident or personal emergency, EAPs can mobilize resources to support *affected employees* and help them cope with the situation.

5. Referrals and Resources: EAPs maintain extensive networks of professionals and resources. They can connect employees with specialists in a variety of fields, from mental health experts to *financial advisors*. This ingenuity ensures employees receive *the specific support* they need to have.

Section 3: Employee Assistance Programs and *Organizational Benefits*

EAPS not only benefits *individual employees*, but also contributes to *the overall health* and success of the organization. When employees are mentally and emotionally well, they are more engaged, productive and satisfied with their work.

Insights:

1. Improved Productivity: Employees who have access to EAPs are more likely to remain productive, even during difficult times. By addressing *personal issues and stressors, they can better focus on their tasks and contribute to the success of the organization.*

2. Reduced Absenteeism and Turnover: EAPs can help reduce employee absenteeism and turnover rates. When employees have the support they need to tackle *personal challenges* , they are more likely to commit to their work.

3. Improved employee morale: Knowing that their employer cares about their well-being can boost employee morale. *A supportive workplace* promotes a sense of loyalty and dedication among staff.

4. Cost Savings: Although implementing EAPs may involve a financial investment, the long-term benefits far outweigh the costs. Lower turnover, increased productivity, and lower healthcare costs due to improved *mental health* all contribute to *significant cost savings*.

5. Competitive Advantage: Organizations that offer comprehensive EAPs can use them as a competitive advantage in attracting and retaining top talent. *Potential employees* are more likely to choose an employer who prioritizes their well-being.

Employee assistance programs are a valuable resource that addresses the complex interplay between work and personal life, ultimately creating a healthier and more productive work environment. These programs underscore the idea that caring for employee *mental health* is not only compassionate, but also a strategic necessity in *the modern workplace*.

CHAPTER TWENTY

Improving community well-being .

1. *Holistic Approaches* to Health and Wellness:

- **Nuance**: the well-being of the community goes beyond mere *physical health* . It includes mental, emotional and social aspects. *A holistic approach* recognizes that these dimensions are interconnected.

- **Perspective 1: Public health professionals**:

- Public health experts emphasize preventive measures, health education and access to health care services. They advocate for policies that address *social determinants* of health, such as housing, education and employment.

- Example: A community health fair that offers free screenings for diabetes, blood pressure, and *mental health* awareness workshops.

- **Perspective 2: social scientists**:

- Social scientists emphasize the role of social networks, community cohesion and social capital in promoting well-being. Strong social bonds can buffer against stress and improve mental health.

- Example: a neighborhood gardening club that promotes *social connections* while promoting physical activity and *healthy eating* .

- **Perspective 3: *Urban Planners and Architects***:

- These professionals shape the built environment. Walk able neighborhoods, *green spaces* and *safe streets* contribute to physical activity and *mental relaxation*.

- Example: a city redesigning its streets to accommodate pedestrians, cyclists and *green spaces*.

- **Perspective 4: Community Leaders and Advocates**:

- *Local leaders play a critical role* in advocating for policies that prioritize health. They engage community members, raise awareness and mobilize resources.

- Example: a grassroots campaign to ban smoking in *public parks, led by concerned citizens.*

- **Perspective 5: Companies and employers**:

- Companies can improve community well-being through workplace wellness programs, flexible work arrangements and supporting *local health initiatives.*

- Example: A technology company that offers gym memberships, mental *health* counseling, and healthy office *snacks.*

2. **Tackling health disparities:**

- **Nuance**: Not all communities have equal access to health care or resources. Health inequalities persist due to socio-economic factors, discrimination and *historical inequality.*

- **Perspective 1: Equality advocates** :

- Advocates emphasize the need to address systemic barriers. They call for targeted interventions to uplift *marginalized communities*.

- Example: a mobile clinic that provides healthcare in *underserved neighborhoods*.

- **Perspective 2: *Cultural competence*** :

- Understanding cultural nuances is crucial. Healthcare providers must tailor their services to *various population groups*.

- Example: *a bilingual health education program* for immigrant families.

- **Perspective 3: Community Health Workers**:

- These frontline workers bridge the gap between healthcare systems and communities. They provide education, navigation and support.

- Example: a community health worker who helps *older residents* manages *chronic conditions*.

3. **Promoting** *an active lifestyle*:

- **Nuance**: physical activity is essential for health. Community design, recreational spaces and *active transportation options* influence behavior.

- **Perspective 1: Parks and Recreation Departments**:

- These departments create *safe parks*, trails and sports facilities. They host fitness classes and community events.

- Example: a city-sponsored program " *Zumba in the Park* ".

- **Perspective 2: Schools and education systems** :

- Schools play a crucial role in shaping children's habits. Physical education, nutritious meals and *active commuting* are important.

- Example: a school that promotes walking or cycling to school through 'Walk to *School Wednesdays* '.

- **Perspective 3: workplace wellness initiatives**:

- Employers can encourage physical activity during working hours. Walking meetings, standing desks, and fitness challenges promote *healthier habits.*

- Example: a company that organizes a lunch walking group.

4. **Mental health support and awareness:**

- **Nuance**: Mental health is an integral part of overall well-being. Reducing stigma, providing resources and promoting resilience are essential.

- **Perspective 1: community-based *mental health* care**:

- Local clinics, support groups and help lines provide *essential help* . They destigmatize seeking help.

- Example: A community center that hosts a depression support group.

- **Perspective 2: Schools and youth programs** :

- Early intervention is important. Schools can teach coping skills, mindfulness and emotional intelligence.

- Example: school counselor leading mindfulness sessions for students.

- Perspective 3: *Mental Health* **Programs in the Workplace**:

- Employers can promote *mental health* days, employee assistance programs and stress management workshops.

- Example: A company that offers *confidential* employee counseling services.

In summary, strengthening community health and well-being requires cross-sector collaboration and tailored approaches

www.ingramcontent.com/pod-product-compliance
Lightning Source LLC
Chambersburg PA
CBHW071216240526
45470CB00018B/1895